Coc

Ketogenic
Diet

Conquer Alzheimer's Disease, Dementia, Mild Cognitive Impairment, and Memory Loss

William Gregory L. Harrison

<u>Disclaimer Notice:</u>
Please note the information contained within this document is for educational and entertainment purposes only. Every attempt has been made to provide accurate, up to date and reliable complete information. No warranties of any kind are expressed or implied. Readers acknowledge that the author is not engaging in the rendering of legal, financial, medical or professional advice. The content of this book has been derived from various sources. Please consult a licensed professional before attempting any techniques outlined in this book.

By reading this document, the reader agrees that under no circumstances are is the author responsible for any losses, direct or indirect, which are incurred as a result of the use of information contained within this document, including, but not limited to, —errors, omissions, or inaccuracies.

WAIT! Before you continue... Are you concerned about your cholesterol and you want to lower it with a proper diet?

If you said yes, then this is your lucky day. I have been searching for simple tips on lowering cholesterol and I've found one great book about it. And right now you can get **FREE ACCESS** for it!

Type this link in your browser to access the book:

http://willglharrison.subscribemenow.com

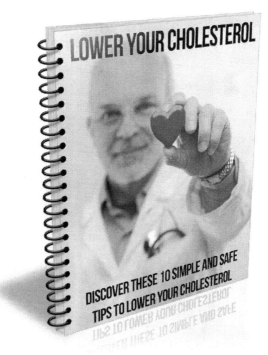

Table of Contents

Introduction

Before you start this book ask yourself these questions:

What do you know about diets and the ketogenic diet?

What do you know about coconuts and the ketogenic diet?

Are you worried about Alzheimer's disease?

This book will tell you about diets and it will explain what a ketogenic diet is in a simple yet factual way that does not blind the reader with science.

It will tell you about coconuts and why they should be part of a ketogenic diet.

Most importantly this book will tell you about Alzheimer's disease and give hope to those worried about this affliction.

It will do this without making false promises.

In this book I will cover diets, the ketogenic diet, coconuts, Alzheimer's disease, scientific research, claims of success, warnings, menus, and recipes. Each chapter will provide a stepping-stone to further exploration if so desired.

Chapter 1: Ketogenic Diet- Health Benefits and Dangers

What is a diet?

A diet is a schedule of eating and drinking where the types and amounts of foods and drinks consumed are formulated to reach a goal. Often diets are part of a commercial program, such as Weight Watchers. Other diets may be part of a religion or social function.

Types of diets

There are many diets. They have all sorts of purposes: control weight, reduction of cholesterol, improving health, etc. Among the diets receiving much publicity are: the Paleo diet, the Mediterranean diet, the Blue Zone diet, the Ornish Diet, the South Beach diet, the Vegan diet, and the list goes on. This book will deal with a diet called the Ketogenic diet, particularly including coconuts.

Preliminary

There are some terms repeatedly used in this book, which the reader may not comprehend very well.

First is *fat*. Fat is a chemical. Some people think that fat is the flab of overweight people. That is only part of the story. Fats are very important chemicals. Fats are scientifically identified as triesters of glycerol and fatty acids. Fat is absolutely crucial for many body functions. Fat gives us energy and enables other foods to carry out their roles. Foods with large amounts of fat include dairy products like cheese and butter, meat, avocados and other fruits, various fishes...the list is almost endless.

Next is *protein*. This has a good reputation. Protein is made of *amino acids*. It is the means by which muscles, bones, skin and other parts of the body are built up. Foods with a large proportion of protein include chicken, meat, dairy products like cheese and butter, fish, soy, and some vegetables.

Last is *carbohydrate*. It is another important part of the diet. The carbohydrates are comprised of a lot of *sugars,* which are converted to glucose during digestion. Carbohydrates supply energy. These foods contain a lot of carbohydrates: pasta, flour, bread, sugary drinks such as the fizzy drinks, fruit juice, and even some vegetables.

What is a ketogenic diet?

Ketogenic diets have been around for a while. In the early twentieth century, it was found they were very effective in the treatment of epilepsy, however, when other treatments for epilepsy were found they were used no longer for this.

In more recent times this diet has been rediscovered and used extensively. It has become very popular on the Internet. There are many sites about it, with some advancing claims, which are at the least questionable.

Basically, a ketogenic diet is a diet with a high fat component, a medium protein component, and a low carbohydrate component.

Why the Ketogenic Diet?

Ketogenic diets have high percentages of fats, moderate percentages of protein, and low percentages of carbohydrates; the purpose of this is for the body to produce chemicals called *ketones*, in the liver, for energy. When a food high in carbohydrates is consumed then the body produces glucose and insulin. Glucose is a chemical that has the easiest molecule for the body to use as energy. It is selected in preference to other energy sources when available.

The body tissues are forced to take glucose from the blood by insulin, and convert it to glycogen stored in the muscles and liver. Fat is stopped by insulin from use as an energy source. If the primary energy source is glucose then your fats are unnecessary in that capacity and are stored in the body.

With a diet that is high in carbohydrates, the body uses glucose as the main energy source. When the intake of carbohydrates is reduced, the body moves into *ketosis*. Ketosis occurs when food intake is changed in this manner. In ketosis, ketones result from the breakdown of fats in the liver. They replace glucose as the energy source.

The aim of ketogenic diets is to put the body into ketosis. Many diets need their clients to spend much time counting calories. Success, or otherwise, depends on these diets having a large decrease in calories. This is not a major feature of ketogenic diets, although there is some calorie counting.

The main aim of the ketogenic diet is realized by the reduction of carbohydrates. The human body is very good at adapting to what it takes in as nourishment. If there is much fat, with only a few carbohydrates, it will use ketones as the principal source of energy.

What happens in ketosis?

This process is very complicated. If the diet has many carbohydrates then glucose levels rise causing the pancreas to release insulin, resulting in glucose going to the body's cells as the energy source. A ketogenic diet causes glucose levels to fall. The pancreas releases *lipase* to be used in the breakdown of fats to *triglycerides*, which go to the liver to be changed to ketones for energy use.

Are there benefits from being in ketosis?

There are numerous benefits. Here are some of them:

- The body's ability to utilize fats as fuel improves. Without this ability, the body is a dependent on a high-carbohydrate diet for energy. In ketosis, it is essential for the body to adapt to using fats as its energy supply.

- Under ketosis, protein is saved for other purposes than energy production. When in ketosis, the body utilizes ketones instead of glucose and hence it is unnecessary for protein to generate glucose as the body has ample supplies of fat.

- The quantity of insulin in the body is lessened. Beneficial hormones are released into the body when insulin levels are reduced.

- The state of ketosis, when combined with increased protein intake, seems to reduce hunger. This is an important benefit for those who wish to lose weight. Diets high in carbohydrate increase hunger. Eating a candy, full of sugar, seems to remove hunger pangs, however, they soon return. Hunger is reduced on a ketogenic diet and satisfied more readily.

Are there dangers to being in ketosis?

On average the positives of the ketogenic diet far outweigh the negatives; however before you start on a ketogenic diet or any other diet, discuss your reasons with your doctor. Here are some possible problems:

- When beginning a ketogenic diet the body has to adapt to changes in metabolism. During this time, a person could be light headed, tired, and thirsty. As soon as the body is using ketones as the principal energy source, it is more energetic than before. It doesn't have the low-blood-sugar crashes that high-carbohydrate meals cause. It is always sensible for those on this diet, and everyone, to drink copious amounts of water.

- The blood-lipid profile is a common way to check. With someone on a ketogenic diet, such a check could cause concern, as a result of a large amount of saturated fat being consumed. Blood-lipid profiles are a source of much controversy; some people on a ketogenic diet have a drop in cholesterol levels, while others have increased cholesterol levels. Cholesterol levels, if increasing are not always bad.

- The reduction in carbohydrates in ketogenic diets could cause deficiency problems in minerals and vitamins. Thiamin, magnesium, iron, calcium, folate, and potassium are sometimes too low in ketogenic diets. Vitamin supplements can help this deficiency.

- The deliberate lowering of carbohydrates could cause a lowering of roughage in the diet resulting in constipation. Bad breath could occur, which has the same cause. These troubles can be overcome with fiber supplements.

- The increase in the quantity of ketones in the body when someone is on a ketogenic diet could cause serious health problems if you are diabetic. Make sure you discuss any ketogenic diet with your doctor before beginning. Generally, though the body can easily able to cope with this diet and reap its benefits.

Chapter 2: Ketogenic Diet with Coconuts

Background

When you say 'coconuts ' a mental picture of tropical paradise in the South Seas or Caribbean and relaxation in tropical resorts is formed.

Coconuts grow on the coconut tree of which they are the fruit. Coconuts are common in tropical climates. They are found in the United States, growing in Hawaii and the southern tip of Florida.

In the wild, the coconut tree usually grows close to the sea. The nuts float on the sea or ocean until coming ashore and germinating.

The coconut is a shallow rooted tree. Fully grown they can reach heights up to 100 feet (30 m). A coconut tree usually produces up to sixty nuts a year. Coconuts are important to many cultures and are very important commercially in the modern world. Most commercial coconut comes from Indonesia or the Philippines.

Wikipedia, the online encyclopedia, describes coconut oil as the edible oil extracted from the kernel or meat of mature coconuts (copra) harvested from the coconut palm. The oil is extracted in a variety of ways from the raw kernel or meat.

Coconut water

Coconut oil is a marvelous product but it must not be confused with coconut water or juice. This comes from young nuts and has a part in the reproduction of the coconut. It is drunk very widely and is frequently served in tropical hotels as a refreshing, non-alcoholic drink.

It is highly effective at rehydration and is very useful for those running long distances, both in training or competition. There are reports where it has been given intravenously due to the absence of a saline solution. This is not usually recommended due to the risk of elevating calcium and potassium levels.

Coconut oil and its history as a food

Coconuts and their oil have been used as a food by human beings for thousands of years. It is used in the food of many regions, including the South Pacific countries, Asia, Central and South American countries, and all parts of Africa where there are coconuts.

For a number of decades in the last century in the West, it was regarded as a source of saturated fat and had its consumption discouraged. Many scientists and health authorities are now questioning this in the light of new evidence.

Coconut oil: its beneficial constituents

Coconut oil unlike other vegetable oils such as corn, olive, peanut, and soybean has a much higher percentage of *saturated, fatty acids*. These also have the name *medium chain triglycerides* (MCTS). Coconut oil has all four MCTS. The main fatty acid in coconut oil is *lauric acid*. The quantity of lauric acid in coconut oil is much higher than in any other vegetable oil. It is very easy to digest the MCTS of coconut oil.

There are still many health authorities advising against a high ingestion of these. However, there is much evidence to show that the type of these found in coconut oil is very beneficial. As you read this book you will repeatedly see that in the field of nutrition expert opinion is much divided.

Human beings are in great need of saturated fat in their diet; many of the dietary problems causing trouble in modern society arise from the bad publicity given to saturated, fatty acids, which are very important in the human diet.

Coconut oil and its history as a traditional medicine

As well as the use of coconuts and their oil as food, the use of the oil as a medicine also goes back thousands of years. Many countries have used coconut oil as a medicine. In India, Ayurvedic medicine (the traditional system of medicine used for that vast country), often used coconut oil. The oil was used for skin problems such as eczema and psoriasis, respiratory conditions, back, shoulder and other joint pains, even problems of the brain. The oil was seen as a remedy for most complaints in Nigeria and some other African countries. In Jamaica and other Caribbean countries, the drinking of coconut oil was seen as a tonic of great benefit. In many South Pacific countries, coconut oil was used as medicine in numerous ways including the relief of pain.

Coconut, its oil, and their benefits

Many benefits are claimed for the use of coconuts and coconut oil, among them:

- Coconut and its oil play an important part in many dishes and recipes;

- Coconut oil can be used as a moisturizer, a hair conditioner and numerous other cosmetic uses;

- Coconut oil is credited by many in helping to lose weight;

- Coconut oil is great for oral health;

- Coconut oil helps digestion;

- Coconut oil is great for relieving stress;

- Coconut oil slows down the aging process;

- Coconut oil is helpful to people suffering from Alzheimer's disease. This book will spend a lot of time examining this;

There are other benefits claimed however the list above is quite amazing. Some items in the list are very important as they indicate possible lines of research and inquiry for those battling some of the most pressing problems bedeviling humanity.

A ketogenic diet encourages the body to rely less on sugar-based fuels and more on fat and ketones for fuel. Ketogenic diets are much easier to attain and adjust with coconuts and their oil. Ketogenic diets need most of the body's energy obtained from fat and no other food provides fat of the quality required, as do coconuts and their oil.

Chapter 3: Beating Alzheimer's, Dementia and Related Diseases with the Coconut Ketogenic Diet

What is Alzheimer's disease?

Alzheimer' disease is a progressive deterioration of the brain that usually happens in middle or old age. It is always fatal and is usually irreversible. It is the most frequent cause of dementia. Alzheimer's is a type of dementia that plays havoc with thinking, memory, and behavior. The symptoms are quite insidious and usually develop slowly, but gets worse and worse over time, to the extent that victims cannot perform basic, daily tasks. Famous people who have had Alzheimer's include the great US president Ronald Reagan, and the popular singer Glenn Campbell.

Alzheimer's was first discovered in 1906, which means that scientists have had a century to find a cure. However, despite their best efforts, there are still no real, universally accepted treatments. Since 2000, there have been more than 200 drugs for Alzheimer's tested and not one has proved to be a silver bullet. Only a few of these drugs in best-case scenarios relieve the memory loss and confusion, which characterizes this dreadful condition.

In the US, one-third of Americans over the age of 85 are already affected by Alzheimer's. In the world, there are nearly 50 million people living with dementia, most of which is Alzheimer's, and without drugs or other treatments, the number affected will double every 22 years. The problem of caring for them will fall to love ones and special facilities. The cost of that care is rapidly mounting, in three years the global annual cost could reach over $1 trillion!

What is Dementia?

Alzheimer's and dementia are often confused. Alzheimer's is a form of dementia. If you have Alzheimer's you have dementia but if you have dementia you do not always have Alzheimer's. Dementia is a term for a set of symptoms that includes impaired thinking and memory loss. Dementia can have causes other than Alzheimer's. Other causes of dementia are Huntington's disease, Parkinson's disease, and Creutzfeldt-Jakob disease.

What causes Alzheimer's?

The cause of Alzheimer's is unknown. What is known is that people affected by Alzheimer's have sticky, plaques of *amyloid* in the brain. Whether this is the cause or an effect of

Alzheimer's is undecided. Another chemical associated with Alzheimer's is *tau*. Tau is a protein, which is often found in the brains of people affected by Alzheimer's.

Is there an accepted cure for Alzheimer's?

Alzheimer's has been successfully cured in mice! Unfortunately, this cure has not yet worked in humans. Most attempts at finding a drug for Alzheimer's have focused on amyloids. Others have been directed at tau and still others at inflammation of the brain. The remainder of this book will be devoted to the relief and reversal of this vile affliction by use of the coconut ketogenic diet.

It is well known know that a poor diet is a major cause of weight gain, heart disease, and diabetes. However, the brain is affected by diet as much as the waistline. Indeed Alzheimer's has been called diabetes of the brain.

In the same way, as a healthy diet can help remove unwanted pounds, it can also stop memory loss. Giving the brain the nutrients it requires improves the memory and halts the development of dementia, which includes Alzheimer's.

It was indicated in an earlier chapter that there has been and is currently a great deal of research into a cure for Alzheimer's disease. A cure has been found which works in mice but not in humans. Some of the research has been on dietary approaches. A particularly interesting investigation is described in the next few paragraphs.

This study, published online in 2016, investigated whether brain energy deficit is a precursor to Alzheimer's. The scientists involved in the study gave four reasons for pursuing this line of research. One of these reasons was the declining brain glucose supply in those at risk of getting Alzheimer's.

This includes people in the '65 and over' age group, even those who are cognitively healthy. This decline can be combated with ketones as the brain's energy supply. Indeed there is evidence to suggest that ketones are the preferred energy source for the brain. The paper discussed various supplements, which can be administered to boost the availability of ketones. It mentioned that the medium chain fatty acids were present in coconut and palm kernel oil, and the supplements needed to increase ketones could be obtained from these[1].

Another study by the same scientists showed that the uptake of ketones to the brain was not negatively correlated with increasing age, as is the uptake to the brain of glucose$_2$.

Other studies also show a ketogenic diet can resist and even overcome symptoms of memory loss and cognitive failure through all the stages of dementia [3-5].

An ideal diet to combat Alzheimer's is as follows:

- Remove all starchy carbohydrates, sweeteners, and grains from the diet.

- Limit the amount of fruit eaten, and eat berries mainly, as their sugar is lower and their antioxidants higher than in other fruits.

- Eat only enough protein for daily needs. If you can then use protein from high-quality sources such as grass-fed meats, freshly caught fish and free-range eggs. Dairy proteins may not be ideal for optimum brain health.

- Eat enough non-starchy vegetables.

- Eat sufficient dietary fats to stop hunger and maintain energy. It is false that animal fats are not healthy for the brain. These are the fats found in meats, fish, and eggs. Stay away from hydrogenated fats (margarine, donuts.), corn oil, sunflower oil, soy oil, and canola. Replace with olive oil and particularly coconut oil.

There are many testimonials to the efficacy of coconuts oil and a ketogenic diet in assisting those with Alzheimer's disease.

The first case is quite well known. Dr. Mary Newport is a successful US doctor whose husband had had Alzheimer's for a number of years. She became certain that diet had an important part to play in this. Dr. Newport's husband was a very capable man but about five years earlier the simple tasks that he could easily do in the past became very difficult.

In her search for a cure, Dr. Newport came across a therapy, which involved MCT (medium chain triglycerides). Dr. Newport's husband was scheduled to have a test soon after her discovery of this therapy; in this test, his Alzheimer's was diagnosed as severe. She got some coconut oil on the way home from the test and started him on it. His improvement was amazing.

Mr. V. Parmar was a 67-year-old process worker in London and had Alzheimer's so badly he didn't even score in the standard test that Alzheimer's sufferers are given. This man's son heard an Oxford University professor of biochemistry extol the possible benefits of coconut oil as a therapy for Alzheimer's so he decided to give his father a couple of teaspoons of the oil twice a day. Since these doses began, Mr. Parmar greatly improved over the period of a year. He is now able to do many activities, which were unthinkable for him a year earlier.

In another case, the wife of a man in Newfoundland Canada had lived a very full and useful life, both with her family and as a secretary. Unfortunately, she got Alzheimer's, nevertheless; her husband heard about the experiences of Dr. Newport and started giving her coconut oil with toast and jam. Since her change of diet, she has greatly improved.

The final testimonial to the efficacy of coconut oil involves a woman who was suffering such bad memory loss and brain fog that she could not even have a conversation with anyone else. Her daughter informed her about coconut oil. The woman has been using it for over a year and is delighted with the results. The fog went away and she is able to drive safely again. She has been able to resume all of her hobbies such as knitting, and crochet, as she is now able to remember patterns again.

The biggest obstacle facing coconut ketogenic diet therapy for Alzheimer's is the lack of a large formal investigation whose results have been peer reviewed. One expert who thinks that this investigation should proceed is Rudy Tanzi, the director of the Genetics and Aging research unit at Massachusetts General Hospital and a professor of neurology at Harvard Medical School. In an article, he explained why coconuts oil could work. 'Virgin coconut oil contains fats that can be converted into ketone which could serve as an alternative energy source for the brain. They could potentially provide energy to the glucose-deprived brains of Alzheimer's sufferers'. He stressed that as yet there is no evidence and warned that coconut oil itself has its own downsides.

There already is a patented supplement, Axona, which is made with coconut oil and which is licensed. Nestle, the large food company, has bought a stake in the manufacturer of this and is planning the sort of large trial that if successful could get Axona a drug license. This would be very helpful in getting it funded as a cure.

In Britain, most experts are skeptical of the coconut oil claims. Professor Robert Howard's of the South London and Maudsley NHS Foundation Trust warned that Alzheimer's has a large placebo reaction. He pointed out that there are times when things seem to be improving and that it is a remitting and relapsing disease. He felt that it is important to protect patients from false hope and quackery. He was not sure that there is a problem with glucose getting into the brain. He thought existing diabetes drugs like Metformin would be better than coconut oil. He pointed out that all manner of things could help patients feel better: music, massage, having a kitten. If people believe coconut oil improves symptoms it probably doesn't do any harm.

The Alzheimer's Society which just had its research funding boosted by the government says it would not discourage anyone from taking coconut oil or ketones but there is not enough evidence to suggest that they have benefits for people with Alzheimer's so they would not consider funding research into it.

David Smith, professor of pharmacology at the physiology institute at Oxford University and director of Optima (Oxford Project to investigate memory and aging), said that this is a mistake. He believes that as a result of the Alzheimer's crisis facing us it's important to have a proper trial.

In summary, it seems that there are experts who are in favor of a conservative approach to the use of the coconut ketogenic diet, and those who give it their qualified support. If you are in a situation involving Alzheimer's it is probably worth trying the coconut ketogenic diet as so-called expert opinion seems to be hopelessly divided.

Chapter 4: Menus and Recipes

What are the features of a ketogenic diet?

The main feature of the ketogenic diet is a high proportion of fat, medium proportion of protein, and a low proportion of carbohydrates. The ratio should be around 11:5:3 however the ratio does not have to be exact as long as you have high fat and low carbohydrates.

What carbohydrates should be used?

Macronutrients are energy sources. Carbohydrates are a macronutrient food type made of sugars, fiber, and starches. They are called carbohydrates, as their molecules are carbon, hydrogen, and oxygen. They are in cake, bread, flour etc., also in fruit and vegetables. Some carbohydrates are good and some are bad:

- The good ones are low to medium in energy; high in nutritional value (minerals, vitamins); natural fiber is high; there is no refined sugar(s) and grain; they are low in sodium;

- The bad ones are high in energy; high in refined sugar(s) and grain; low in fiber; low in nutritional value; high in sodium.

What protein should be used?

Protein, like carbohydrate, is a macronutrient. It is a source of energy. It is essential for the repair and building of muscles. Around 15% of the mass of the human body is protein. Protein is made of chemicals called amino acids. These are comprised of carbon, hydrogen, oxygen, sulfur and nitrogen. You find protein in poultry, meat, fish, eggs, nuts and beans. Your meals should include them.

What fats should be used?

Fats are macronutrients and are essential in nutrition. Without fat life is impossible. Fat is full of energy. There are higher concentrations of energy in fat than in the same quantities of either protein or carbohydrates. The best fats are found in butter, virgin olive oil, avocado oil, and particularly coconut oil.

Diet Aids

Very useful devices to help you, when on a ketogenic diet, are calorie counters. This measures the quantity of energy used by the diet. A number websites have good calorie counters. These are easily be found by Googling 'online calorie counter'.

A good one for finding your needs is www.mydreamshape.com/daily-calorie-needs-calculator. One with the calorie contents of seemingly all foods is www.fitwatch.com/caloriecounter

Ketogenic Diet for Alzheimer's

Here is a diet based on the need for a weight loss of 2 lb. a week for a woman of age 64. She weighs 280 lb. and leads a sedentary life. She is obviously very obese and, particularly at her age should lose a lot of weight. She is a prime candidate for Alzheimer's.

According to a calorie counter, her daily calorie intake should be 1291 calories.

For one day

Food	Meal	Qty.	Calories	Fat
Ground Meat	Breakfast	4 ounces	250	160
Onion	Breakfast	1 ounce	45	32
Milkshake with coconut oil	Breakfast	1 glass	200	100
Piece of oily fish such as cod	Lunch	1	100	30
Cauliflower	Lunch	1 serving	150	90

Salad with dressing	Lunch	1 serving	70	40
Pork chop	Dinner	1	220	90
Spinach	Dinner	2 cups	41	5
Salad with dressing	Dinner	1 serving	70	40
		Total	**1146**	**587**

The value of 1146 is well within the calorie limit of 1291 so she could increase the foods and/or amounts. If she is a wine drinker then she should not have a glass of wine as each glass has about 120 calories, and if she is following a ketogenic diet these would not be good. Each glass of wine has no fat and on a ketogenic diet, the idea is to maximize fat intake. If the percentage of calories from fat is calculated it will be found to be a bit more than 51.2%. Cooking the spinach and fish in coconut oil can easily increase this. Keeping track of calories becomes much simpler as you get familiar with it.

What's for Breakfast?

Breakfast is the first meal of the day. It should be consumed no more than two hours after arising and it should be treated as important. It has to keep you going during a most important part of the day.

Smoothies

For those in a rush, the smoothie is a real timesaver. A smoothie is a drink obtained by mixing liquids and solid in a blender. For the many who are at best only tolerant of vegetables, these can be put into smoothies, particularly if you have a blender.

For those on a ketogenic diet for the maximum nutritional benefit, you could use any or all of coconut milk, yogurt, nuts, avocado, chocolate, turmeric, coconut oil, and sometimes food supplements like protein powder. There are thousands of smoothie recipes on the Internet. Go to Google and type in 'How do you make a ketogenic smoothie'.

If you haven't got a blender then you can use a whisk, juicer or eggbeater. It is best, though, if you can afford one, to get a good blender as you can really experiment with smoothies until you find one that is ideal for you.

Muesli

This is a form of cereal, usually quite expensive, and loaded with carbohydrates. Even if you make your own, unless you restrict the ingredients to nuts (almonds, walnuts, macadamia), chia seed, linseed, yogurt it is probably not a good addition to breakfast.

Cooking
The process of cooking tends to slow things down and if you're in a hurry you may decide that you won't do any cooking. The use of a microwave is a great help if you want some hot food for breakfast. Here are some suggestions:

Porridge
This is a great breakfast food. Unfortunately, the carbohydrate content of porridge is high, nonetheless you can replace oatmeal porridge with flax meal if you really want porridge.

Another marvelous and delicious addition to breakfast that can be made very quickly is an omelet.

Omelet
Get the following ingredients: Three whole eggs (include yolks), four ounces (100g) of mincemeat or other diced meat, an ounce of grated cheese, pepper, two tablespoons of coconut oil. Mix the ingredients meticulously. Microwave thoroughly at a high temperature for a minute. Stir then microwave at that temperature for another minute. Take out of the microwave and allow to cool. This is a very nutritious little meal, which is quickly prepared.

Beverages
Coffee has received a lot of criticism over the years. Consumption of it has been linked with a number of physical complaints and problems. Fortunately, in more recent times, it has been realized that, in moderation, it poses no threat to health at all. The only qualification, might be, is that it is best to avoid sugar as a sweetener. The same comments can be placed alongside tea, another very widely drunk beverage. The best types of tea to drink are herbal and these are always best with no additives.

Fruit juice has a lot of sugar, particularly commercial juices. Best to have a smoothie, coffee or tea if on a ketogenic diet.

What's for Lunch?
Lunch is a meal eaten near the middle of the day. Often lunch is the second, major meal of the day after breakfast. It can vary in size depending on need, and possibly culture. It is important for maximum efficiency to take a break near the middle of the day, have something to eat and catch your breath.

Wholegrain sandwiches and pasta?
The value of a healthy breakfast was emphasized and the same applies to lunch. You must have enough energy for the afternoon.

The lunch of those not on a ketogenic diet often consists of sandwiches, rolls, wraps etc. that are all full of carbohydrates.

Grain substitutes can be made by using finely chopped broccoli or cauliflower instead of grain. When combined with cheese and other protein sources and fried with coconut oil a ketogenic pizza is possible, similarly, avocados and zucchinis can be used as 'boats'. There are numerous references to these by Googling 'avocado ketogenic boat' or 'zucchini ketogenic boat'.

Pizza

The ingredients for a pizza usually have too many carbohydrates in them however it is possible to make a pizza base, which is suitable for a ketogenic diet. Here is a good one.

The ingredients are:

- 2 cups of mozzarella cheese (you could try any grated cheese)
- three-quarters of a cup of almond flour (you could try coconut flour)
- 1 tablespoon of psyllium husk powder to provide roughage
- 3 tablespoons of cream cheese
- one large egg
- 1 tablespoon of Italian seasoning
- half a teaspoon of salt
- half a teaspoon of pepper

Instructions:

1. Preheat the oven to 400°F, while this is being done measure out the mozzarella cheese and put it into a microwave bowl;
2. Add the three-quarters of a cup of almond flour, the psyllium husk powder, the Italian seasoning, the half a teaspoon of salt and the half a teaspoon of pepper;
3. Thoroughly mix until it is a ball;

4. Cover it with 1 tablespoon of coconut oil to make it easy to work with;
5. Spread the bowl on baking paper;
6. Put in the pre-warmed oven;
7. Bake the spread out pizza for 10 minutes on one side;
8. Remove the pizza from the oven;
9. Flip it over and bake for another 2 to 4 minutes:
10. Remove it from the oven and cover it with a topping (as an example you could use half a cup of tomato sauce, 1 cup of mozzarella cheese and some slices of pepperoni); and
11. Allow to cool, cut sit into slices then eat.

Salads
Salads are a very healthy lunch food. Make sure that you use vegetables, which go with a ketogenic diet. Such vegetables are kale, spinach, lettuce, broccoli, zucchini, cucumbers, and cauliflowers. Avoid potatoes, peas, beans, and corn as they are high in carbohydrates.

Salads can include chicken, cheese or tuna. These provide protein, essential to the repair of the body. Fish can also be included; the omega-3 fatty acids found in mackerel, herring and sardines have been identified as being of great nutritional benefit. Salads can include coconut and coconut oil in the dressing.

Soup
Soup is ideal for lunch for people on the ketogenic diet. It is warming, nutritious and easily put in a vacuum flask for quick use. Many kinds of soup can be made with meat or fish. You can include coconut oil. The preparation time of soup is short which is helpful for busy people.

What's for Dinner?
For most dinner is the most important meal of the day, usually in the evening, but in some countries in the middle of the day. In the English-speaking world, dinner is in the

evenings. We will be considering it in a form suited to the needs of those on a ketogenic diet.

Meat and other protein

Meat and fish are very important in ketogenic diets. They contain plenty of fat, so important to those on this diet. There is an almost limitless variety of them and methods by which they can be prepared. Here is a possible recipe for pork chops:

- Create the base for the pork chops by using coconut flour in a container. Make sure that it's a container that can fit the pork chops;

- Mix with some warm coconut oil, some black pepper, some turmeric powder some cayenne pepper and some salt (you can try all sorts of spices; cloves are nice; so is cinnamon);

- Make sure that both sides of the chops are covered with this mixture when you do that you could cover the pork chops with coconut oil;

- Fry them until they have a nice golden brown color; and

- When this is complete you may take them out and eat them.

This is only one possibility. You can try others as most are delicious, even if you are only experimenting.

Salads
Although highly recommended for lunch; they are also a great addition to your dinner. They are easy to prepare and very nutritious. It is easy to get coconut oil in them, either through the actual addition of coconut, or the inclusion of coconut oil in the dressing.

Vegetables and Beans
These are an important part of most diets but must be carefully dealt with if you're on a ketogenic diet as many are full of carbohydrates. Refer to the comments about vegetables in the section in this chapter on lunch.

Desserts
You may think these have a lot of sugar and not much nutritional value and are not very suitable for a ketogenic diet but they do not have to be. Many people crave sweet food to finish their dinner. There are many desserts, ideal for the ketogenic diet. Google 'desserts for

a ketogenic diet'. You will get endless hits and many of the sites have truly delicious offerings.

Conclusion

A diet is a schedule of meals and food.

A ketogenic diet is a diet whose energy is predominantly provided by fat.
Coconuts and their oil should be part of a ketogenic diet.

Alzheimer's disease is a very serious problem throughout the world.

There is a lot of evidence, both scientific and anecdotal, that a ketogenic diet, which includes coconuts and its oil will help to reduce and even reverse the symptoms of Alzheimer's, dementia, mild cognitive impairment and memory loss.

For most people a ketogenic diet including coconuts and the oil is harmless and worth trying if they wish to prevent or overcome Alzheimer's.

You will have to decide for yourself whether to proceed with one.

References

1. Cunnane, S. C., Courchesne-Loyer, A., Vandenberghe, C., St-Pierre, V., Fortier, M., Hennebelle, M., ... Castellano, C.-A. (2016). Can Ketones Help Rescue Brain Fuel Supply in Later Life? Implications for Cognitive Health during Aging and the Treatment of Alzheimer's disease. *Frontiers in Molecular Neuroscience*, 9, 53. http://doi.org/10.3389/fnmol.2016.00053

2. Cunnane S. C., Courchesne-Loyer A., St-Pierre V., Vandenberghe C., Pierotti T., Fortier M., et al. (2016). Can ketones compensate for deteriorating brain glucose uptake during aging? Implications for the risk and treatment of Alzheimer's disease. *Ann. N. Y. Acad. Sci.* 1367 12–20. 10.1111/nyas.12999

3. A ketogenic diet delays weight loss and does not impair working memory or motor function in the R6/2 1J mouse model of Huntington's disease. Physiol Behav. 2011 Jul 6;103(5):501-7. Epub 2011 Apr 9.

4. Kim DY, Hao J, Liu R, Turner G, Shi F-D, et al. (2012) Inflammation-Mediated Memory Dysfunction and Effects of a Ketogenic Diet in a Murine Model of Multiple Sclerosis. PloS

ONE 7(5): e35476.
Doi:10.1371/journal.pone.0035476.

5. Dietary ketosis enhances memory in mild cognitive impairment. Neurobiology of Aging. Volume 33, Issue 2 , Pages 425.e19-425.e27, February 2012.

I need your help...

Thank you so much for taking the time to finish this book.

But I need your help...

I want to reach as many people as I can to make them aware of the content of this book. One of the best ways to do that is to have many honest reviews about the book. Plus, it will help me assess my book better and revise it if needed, to better suit the needs of my readers.

Hence, if you've gained some insights from this book, would you be so kind to leave a review of this book?

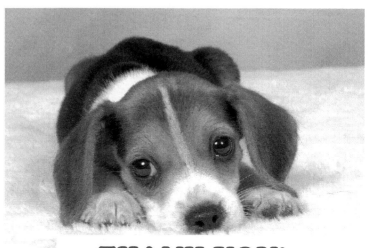

THANK YOU!

Type this URL on the website to redirect you to Amazon.

https://www.amazon.com/dp/B01N5PX W4Y

Again, thank you so much and best wishes!

-William Gregory L. Harrison

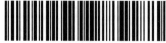

Made in the USA
San Bernardino, CA
16 May 2017